HEALTHY

HOT

HAPPY

Simple Baby Steps to a Better You

By Susan Goddard

This book previously published as...

To Age or Not to Age, That is Your Choice

Publisher:

Model Masters, Inc
297 Kingsbury Grade, Suite.D
Stateline, NV 89449

ISBN: 9798621026318

DEDICATION

This book is dedicated to my loving husband, Bill,who often volunteers as my guinea pig and without whose encouragement and support this book would never have been written.

A Letter to My Readers

> *"Getting older is inevitable;*
> *Aging is optional."*
>
> Dr. Christiane Northrup

I heard Dr. Northrup say this while listening to her online. It really hit a chord with me and I thought how true this statement really was. This one quote inspired me to write this book and share my thoughts with you.

We cannot stop the years from passing but WE CAN keep our body, mind and spirit from what we call 'aging'. By eating the right foods, doing the right exercises including some for our mind, and thinking young instead of 'old', de-stressing and connecting with our spirit we can feel like we're 30 when we are 70!

I wrote this book to be an easy to read tool filled with good information and simple, helpful tips to help you move forward. I am not a medical doctor, do not have a PhD, nor am I a certified nutritionist. What I do have is over 40 years of experience in learning and applying the principles that will be outlined in this book.

I tried to keep this book short enough so it won't take you weeks to read. I also will keep out all the medical jargon and technical terminology that most of us don't understand anyway.

After each chapter I have listed some baby steps to follow. As Martin Luther King, Jr. said "If you can't see the whole staircase just take the first step". First and foremost is to make the commitment to yourself to get healthy. Next, I would encourage you to take the baby steps I recommend. Make one little change at a time and become comfortable with it. Once you've completed that step then take the next one and before you know it you will be to the top of the staircase of vibrant health!

This book is my gift to you. Recently my grandson asked me what my super power would be if I was a superhero. My immediate response was "to make everyone healthy."

My wish is that after reading this book you will realize that you don't have to have declining health, degenerative disease, be overweight and you DO NOT have to age regardless of how many birthdays you've had!

You have the power to take back your life; the ageless, healthy, beautiful YOU.

Enjoy life!

TABLE OF CONTENTS

WHO IS SUSAN GODDARD AND WHY SHOULD I READ THIS BOOK?

As I approached my 65th birthday I finally had to face the reality that I could no longer keep telling everyone that I turned 49 each birthday! But the reality is that I feel like I am in my forties and sometimes I think that I am in better shape now than when I was in my thirties, despite a few wrinkles!

Granted I have not always eaten the healthiest of diets but I tried to do the best I could. I have, however, watched my health as far as listening to signals my body gives me as to what I should and shouldn't be eating or doing, keeping my immune system strong, staying away from as many artificial food additives and preservatives (chemicals) as I could and always researching natural cures for myself and family when one was needed.

I have struggled with my weight since my late twenties; not a lot of weight but 25 pounds over the years was still more than I wanted. Consequently, I have been a yo-yo dieter for over 30 years and no matter how I did on any given diet and kept the weight off for maybe 6 months I always gained it back. I finally have unlocked the key to weight loss and I will tell you all about it in Chapter 7.

I have been studying natural/alternative medicine for over 40 years which also includes eating the right foods for a healthy body and brain. Long before the internet was around I subscribed to many newsletters on this subject and they were all delivered by the mailman! I became so excited when one would arrive in the mail and would read it over and over again.

I still have my collection (actual hard copies) and I still often refer to them. My passion for this stuff grew and I was always testing out what I had learned.

When someone in my household came down with something; allergic reaction, bad cold or cough, back pain, poison ivy, sore throat, and the list goes on…

I would look through all my newsletters and find a natural cure, use it and without fail it worked. This always made me more excited and I had to know more.

Now the next thing I have to say may get me into trouble with a lot of people and pharmaceutical companies but I must say it. Prescription drugs only mask symptoms--they are not a cure. The side effects are far worse than whatever ails you and some can actually be deadly.

You will read in this book why I am so against putting prescription drugs (especially broad spectrum antibiotics for non-bacterial infections) into our bodies and how almost every man, woman and child is now ingesting these drugs through drinking the city tap water making matters worse for an entire population.

Specific antibiotics would be the only prescription drug that is a life saver when you have an actual bacterial infection. They should never be taken for any other reason such as relieving symptoms of a bad cold or flu (neither a bacterial infection but a virus). If you need to take antibiotics, however, it is a very good idea to take probiotics to replenish your gut bacteria because an antibiotic kills indiscriminately, meaning it kills both the good and bad bacteria in your gut. More on that in Chapter 5.

I have not taken any prescription drugs in over 40 years, applied natural and alternative cures when needed and did the best I could eating a healthy diet. I know that following these three things have kept me in excellent health all these years.

In the last year I have been swept up with the vast amount of new discoveries, research and studies on our bodies and brains. I have listened to countless hours of online seminars and interviews, read several books, newsletters and reports, and have done tons of research on health and aging. I have applied what I've learned in my life and the lives of my family and countless friends.

I have accumulated so much knowledge about what we can do to remain in the best health and stay young throughout our lives. Now that I am 65, NOT aging has become one of my top priorities. I realized that writing this book just had to happen. So to all of you who don't want to devote their time to researching every little thing--this book is for you.

For those who have never realized that eating a nutrient rich diet, taking the necessary supplements, using alternative or natural medicine, and feeding your brain the right fats can give you great health, both body and brain, this book's for you.

There are also specific foods that can reverse many of our health issues and even many degenerative diseases. I will go into more of this in later chapters.

I decided to write this book because I want to share my passion and years of experience with my readers. My hope is that by giving you this basic information it will inspire and empower you to learn more and change the way you look at food and the part it plays in living a vibrant, healthy life.

Maybe with this new found knowledge, you can teach and empower your children that a healthy body and mind comes from eating the proper foods and eliminating as many toxins as possible. Then your children can pass this along to the next generations for healthier, happier and longer lives.

Once you become aware of the basic info I put in this book you can always do more research if you wish. The internet is a great place to start but make sure it's from a credible source because there's a lot of junk out there too. Check out the RESOURCES section for a list of some great books on how to cure some of our most prolific diseases like cancer and heart disease just by changing what we eat.

I am not writing this book based just on things I've heard but on my own research, experience and application of these practices. Please read this book with an **open mind** because health and aging really do start there. You can also visit my blog at www.SusanGoddardBlog.com

Get healthy, stay young and live with vigor and happiness everyday while you're still on this planet!

PART ONE

FOOD FOR THOUGHT

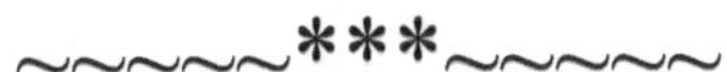

"There are no constraints on the human mind, no walls around the human spirit, no barriers to our progress except those we ourselves erect."

Ronald Reagan

Chapter 1

WHAT MAKES A HEALTHY BRAIN

To start this chapter I would just like to give you some basic information on the brain. . .

This big bundle of nerve cells is mostly gray, white and a little pink and has the texture of tofu! I guess this is why it's called gray matter. It serves as the center of the nervous system.

Weighing in at only 3 pounds it is made up of about 100 billion neurons that gather and transmit signals. The nerve cells can be compared to tiny little wires which actually carry electrical signals. These signals provide the information that tell us how to walk and talk, what we see, feel, smell, what we think and control other bodily functions.

It is more powerful than any computer on earth. Recent research carried out as part of the AI Impacts project found that even today's most advanced supercomputers are only one-thirtieth as powerful as the human brain.

The brain is composed of about 75% water and is the fattiest organ in the body. Consisting of a minimum of 60% fat you can understand how important it is to eat lots of fat to maintain a healthy brain, **but only the good fats**. We sure don't want to starve our brain of what it needs nor do we want to clog it up with unhealthy trans-fats.

Our brain function also has a direct connection to the gut. This makes our gut health extremely important to maintaining a healthy brain. With a balanced flora in our gut and eating the right fats and whole foods we can eliminate memory decline and dementia and increase our learning and concentration capacity.

Could this be the beginning to ending Alzheimer's? Much of the recent scientific research and studies are leaning this way. There is currently no cure for the dreaded Alzheimer's, but as I write this book the simple cure may be as easy as changing your diet to whole foods and good fats.

Feed your brain what it really needs to function properly and this will serve you well. I don't believe that there is an expiration date on our organs as long as we feed them what they need. Eating whole foods and good fats that give our bodies the vitamins, minerals, and amino acids our organs need to function is the best advice I can give to staying young, healthy and sharp as a tack!

Baby Steps for Chapter 1

1. Start cutting out ALL trans-fats and hydrogenated fats from your   diet.

2. Read labels when you shop. Don't buy if it contains either of the above.

3. Slowly take steps to eliminate fried foods from your diet. Just eliminate your least favorite fried food for a month and see how good you'll feel.

Chapter 2

WE ARE PROGRAMMED TO GET OLD

We are pre-programmed by our society that our body and mind starts going downhill sometime after the age of 40. Think about when you were a child…

You often heard grandparents complaining about their aching joints, high cholesterol numbers, forgetting where they put things, being tired all the time and you also noticed how many 'older' people walk hunched over, use a walker or one of the electric scooters.

As children we begin to correlate getting older with all of these symptoms we notice in our elders. We also get bombarded by television commercials about a pill for everything. Mostly older people are shown in these ads, thus, more programming for our brains as to all the ailments we will have as we age.

What we see and hear about on a consistent basis programs our brains to think that as we get older we automatically begin to decline and end up with one or all of the diseases you hear about on TV. However, this is just a perception, yet, it is one we've grown up with.

It is only true if you believe it. Yes, let me say that again…

this is only true if YOU BELIEVE it. Your body is incredible and as long as you take care of it; feed it the proper nutrients it needs, get plenty of sleep (time for repair work), and de-stress your life you can live into your hundreds with vibrant health!

It is true that as we get older the production of many of the hormones that keep us young and vibrant slow down. Also a lifetime of stress has caused your body to produce more of the stress hormones which create all kinds of problems including weight gain. Eating the right foods, not putting toxins and chemicals into your body, mild exercising and meditation (or just relaxing for 30 minutes on a daily basis) can and will keep you in good health throughout the rest of your existence here on earth.

In the following chapters I will present you with many foods you should be eating and many which you should never eat in order to keep yourself healthy and young.

Baby Steps for Chapter 2

1. Mute the prescription commercials that brainwash you into thinking you will get a particular disease when you get older. Better yet, turn off the TV altogether.

2. Do not believe everything you see and hear in any ads.   Advertising is simply a way to make companies money, but they can program your brain if you watch enough commercials.

3. Tell yourself at least once a day that YOU look and feel great, even if you don't really feel that way yet. Remember, baby steps!

Chapter 3

YOUR THOUGHTS CONTROL YOUR LIFE

For the last several years I have been studying the mind which plays a major role in your health and aging because what you **believe** is what you will manifest in your life. Your life is the mirror of your thoughts. In other words, if you constantly think about catching the next cold or flu every month, you will. If you think you look old and feel old, you're aging. This is where we must learn to always think and speak positive to ourselves.

Our thoughts and self-talk are an extremely powerful first step to becoming healthy and staying young. This may sound easy but you must become aware of your thoughts at all times. When you catch yourself stating something in the negative; *"Seems like I catch a cold every month"* STOP, and rephrase it to something positive like; *"I feel strong and healthy and no cold will get the best of me."* Even if you don't believe what you're saying in the moment, keep practicing this and I assure you that you won't be getting a cold every month. Your mind believes what you tell it and that transfers to your body.

There is now a new science of Epigenetics which has proven that your ancestors' genes may be passed down to you but these genes are not necessarily expressed by your body's cells. What this means is that if a family member has some genetic disease you are not doomed with that same disease. Scientists have shown that there are many factors that can switch genes on and off and affect how cells express genes.

Though my idea hasn't been proven yet, I believe that just by *thinking* you will get the disease that your family member has/had you will and if you think you won't get that disease you won't, no matter if 'it runs in the family'. The mind is more powerful than most people realize. It even astonishes the scientists and researchers who are studying the brain.

Yes, everything actually starts in your brain with your thoughts and what you believe creates your reality. If you believe you will have arthritis or clogged arteries when you hit 50 chances are you will.

A longtime friend of mine was always saying things like he would be in a nursing home by the time he was in his fifties or he'd be dead by the time he's 60 so why bother changing his bad habits of smoking and eating unhealthy. I would always discourage him from talking that way but he kept it up. And guess what? Yes, sadly he died of a heart attack at age 59. I believe he had totally convinced his brain that 59 years old was his ultimate doom.

Our minds are very powerful and if this is what you're thinking, this is probably what you'll get. So, I say quit talking or thinking about how stressed you are, or how your joints ache, or how you catch a cold every month. Instead, think and say positive statements about your body and health even when you do have aches and pains. Notice how much healthier you will feel by just telling yourself you feel good.

The brain is one of the most powerful tools in our body, yet we really don't learn how to use it properly. In later chapters we will be going into much more detail about your thinking and what foods your brain needs to stay healthy and fend off Alzheimer's and dementia.

In Chapter 1 I mentioned how our brain sends out electrical signals throughout the body. Well, every time we think a thought the brain sends that signal. So it stands to reason that if you think a good thought the signal coursing through your body from your brain should make you feel good. On the other hand, if you think a negative thought the signal will make you feel bad. This is why it is so very important to be aware of all your thoughts. No matter what is in front of you, try to turn it into a positive thought and *note your success* at doing so. Every time you have a success you will release endorphins, the brain's "feel-good" chemicals, and soon you will be hooked on your many successes.

One more thing on the power of our mind I want to mention; the Placebo Effect. I'm sure you have heard of this and most drug research studies use this as comparisons; what works better, the drug or a placebo (usually a sugar pill with no medication at all). People given a placebo thinking it is a drug for what ails them more often than not have miraculous results. Why is this? Because it all comes down to what their mind <u>believes</u>. When they convince themselves that the pill they are given will cure them it doesn't matter that it's a sugar pill, the mind is more powerful than a pill.

Baby Steps for Chapter 3

1. Become aware of the way you negatively speak or think of yourself by stopping and saying something nice instead.

2. Give yourself compliments and be grateful when you receive them as well.

3. Start patting yourself on the back for each small success (no matter what it is) and see how good it feels.

4. One positive thought at a time adds up to huge results.

PART TWO

FOOD FOR THE BODY

"Let food be thy medicine and medicine

be thy food"

Hippocrates

(Greek physician regarded as the father of
medicine)

Chapter 4

HOW YOUR BODY WORKS

It is your personal responsibility to take care of the body you were given. After all, you can't go to the store and exchange it for another. Disease prevention and curing the underlying problems is what we should be focused on. There is enough knowledge, research, tools and technology to prevent most diseases, yet people seem to ignore their health until it stops them in their tracks. Prevention is the key word here and that rests squarely on your shoulders. Choose to be healthy!

Feeding your body and mind the proper nourishment can keep them running smoothly. When you learn that refined, highly processed foods and sodas are basically nutrient deficient, you must understand why it is so important to eat whole, natural foods to feed your engine.

Our bodies are so complex that every day researchers find out something new about them. What we do know is that our body needs the correct fuel to perform all the functions that keep us alive, repair itself and give us the energy to walk, run and think.

In a way you can compare the body to a car engine. You put fuel (gasoline) into your car to make it go and if you ever got a bad batch of gasoline or ran the tank down too low then you know how the car sputters and eventually stops running. You can't run your car on empty and neither can you run your body that way!

Our body also needs fuel (food). Not just any food will do if you want to be healthy. Whole, natural foods contain the vitamins, minerals, amino acids, etc. that keeps our engine running and in tip top shape.

Every cell in your body needs the proper nutrients and they can only get them from the foods you feed yourself. Our bodies can walk into the grocery store and push a shopping cart but our minds must make the decision on the best foods to be throwing into that cart. So it stands to reason that when you buy foods with no nutritional value, your cells, all 37.2 trillion of them, will slowly begin to run out of energy (like the car running out of gas). In reality you are preventing your cells from doing their job of keeping you healthy and disease free.

If you have not been eating nutritionally for most of your life it will catch up to you sooner or later. You may not notice it right away but as you get older you start to see the deterioration and decline in your health, skin and energy level. If you've already seen and felt some not so good changes in your health there is good news.

There are tons of recent research and studies which prove that you can actually reverse (yes, reverse) many of our most common diseases such as heart disease and certain cancers. Also, many of these studies show that you can prevent many of the most common diseases from ever taking place in your body just by eating the right foods and eliminating chemically processed HFCS (high fructose corn syrup), artificial flavoring and coloring, and other toxins from your diet.

Remember, getting older does not mean your health starts declining and your body and mind start deteriorating *unless you let it.* I will go into more details in later chapters, but for starters I want you to give some serious thought to changing your diet if you are living on chicken nuggets, cheese burgers, French fries and sodas.

What is the right nutrition you ask? Well I am not a nutritionist, therefore, can't really tell you exactly what you should be eating for breakfast, lunch and dinner every day of the year. Through all of my research I can suggest to you some of the very best nutrient rich foods you should definitely be adding to your meal plans.

The Five Foods you must ADD to your meals:

1. Dark leafy greens; kale, spinach, turnip greens, etc.

2. Cruciferous veggies; broccoli, cauliflower, cabbage and there are many more

3. Good fats; Extra virgin coconut or olive oils, avocado, grass fed butter, olives, seeds and tree nuts

4. Berries; blueberries, strawberries, blackberries, etc.

5. Omega 3 fatty acids: from fish, chia seeds, flaxseed oil, walnuts

Bonus; many of the above foods also have <u>anti-aging properties</u>.

The following list shows the most common foods that are problematic for many people.

The Eight Foods you must AVOID:

1. Dairy (substitute with almond, cashew or coconut milk)

2. Peanuts, including peanut butter (substitute with tree nut butters like almond butter)

3. Soybean oil, soy protein isolate; which seems to be in everything these days especially most so called 'protein bars'

4. Sugar and artificial sweeteners (see Chapter 6 for more details)

5. Gluten (over the past 50 years wheat has been hybridized so much that our bodies can no longer metabolize the gluten molecule)

6. Corn (most corn is now genetically modified and it is used to fatten cattle and pigs) Can it be fattening you up too?

7. Eggs (not a problem for many people and you may be okay with eggs but do a test first)
8. Hydrogenated or Partially Hydrogenated fats and oils from Canola, Sunflower, Corn, Soy

The 8 foods listed above should definitely be avoided because many of these foods can cause weight gain, intolerance or sensitivities causing allergy-like symptoms, brain fog, fatigue, skin rashes, breakouts and auto-immune diseases.

The best way to tell if any of the above 8 foods are causing you any problems is to take all eight of these foods out of your diet at once for three weeks. You may start feeling better and many symptoms as mentioned above may disappear. However, if there are any of these foods you can't live without, add one at a time back into your diet. Give it a week or two and see if any symptoms reoccur. If so, you know that your body cannot tolerate that particular food. In that case it is a matter of giving up that food forever or suffering from the symptoms it reveals.

Baby Steps for Chapter 4

1. Become informed (by reading this book) and <u>make a commitment</u> to yourself to eat healthier starting now.

2. Share this information with your family so they can make better decisions as well about what they eat.

3. Add at least 1 food per week from the list of 5 Foods to Add. Try different greens or cruciferous veggies to see which ones you like the best then start adding them every day.

4. Eliminate 1 food per week from the list of 8 Foods to Avoid. For example: switch from cow's milk to cashew milk (my favorite), or maybe you'll like almond milk better. Swap your canola or corn oil for extra virgin coconut oil.

5. Try your best to eventually add all the good foods to your everyday meals and

eliminate the bad ones permanently.
Baby steps add up!

Chapter 5

THE IMPORTANCE OF YOUR GUT

I have devoted a long chapter to the gut because most people have no idea that the gut is **critically important** to your health. There is an old adage that says health begins and ends in the gut. If you were to ask people what the function of their gut is the most common reply would probably be 'to digest your food'. This answer is correct but there is so much more…

Your body only has three direct connections to the outside world: your skin, your respiratory tract and your gut. This makes the gut one of the places most exposed and vulnerable.

There are 100 trillion organisms in your gut which are called your microbiome. This microbiome can be referred to as your 'inner garden'. Your inner garden is a place that you must nurture with nutritious foods and eliminate toxins from entering your body as best you can.

There are three main reasons why gut health is front and center to maintaining a vibrantly healthy mind, body and spirit:

1. It is crucial to your comfort when it comes to gas, bloating, heartburn, constipation and diarrhea

2. 60-70% of your immune system is
   located in the digestive track

3. It plays a critical role in the health of your
   brain, including your mood

I will cover each one of these reasons in further detail on the following pages. By making you aware that many, many health issues can be directly or indirectly related to your gut health you will be empowered to take action (nurture your inner garden) after reading this chapter.

DIGESTION

Most people think of the gut as the system which digests the food and then sends it out the other end. As we will soon learn digestion is only one of the functions of the gut.

When our digestion is working great we don't give it any thought, however, when you're gassy, bloated, constipated or are suffering with heartburn you blame it all on indigestion. These symptoms and more seem to be the norm in our society today. If you watch any television at all the ads for antacids, both over-the-counter and prescription drugs, flood the airwaves.

What causes most of these uncomfortable conditions is more than likely the foods you are eating; one of the biggest being lots of sugar. Unless you have a diet of whole, natural foods your meals are probably laden with sugars in some form or another. You may not even realize this if you don't read labels.

You would be hard pressed to find on grocery store shelves any food (canned or packaged) that does not have some form of sugar in it even if that particular food is not meant to be sweet. Most processed foods today have substituted real sugar for the much sweeter, chemically processed High Fructose Corn Syrup. On food labels you find these HFCS in addition to a list of artificial flavors, colorings and preservatives. Who really knows what they are; I say if you can't pronounce it don't eat it!

These ultra-processed, chemically altered, pre-packaged foods we buy and prepare for our meals are not even real foods. And not being real food they contain nothing that our body needs. As a matter of fact, our body doesn't even know how to process these foods once they enter our system. Our bodies are not chemical factories and cannot digest and assimilate these foreign food-like substances which are mostly devoid of any nutritional value.

If you have any digestive problems as mentioned above it would be a good idea to pay close attention to what foods you are eating. Learn to listen to your body. Symptoms are usually your body's way of telling you something is off…so stop and listen and make a change. Here are four things that may help stop many digestive symptoms before they begin:

- Do not eat while stressed (take 30 seconds to calm yourself before taking that first bite)

- Be sure to chew your food well (your saliva begins the digesting process)

- Get more fiber in your diet

- Stop taking antacids. Your stomach is more than likely <u>not</u> producing enough acid (contrary to what you may think) thus making matters worse.

There is also a common problem today which is called leaky gut syndrome. It is actually named for exactly what it is; a leaky gut. When your gut bacteria are disrupted it may cause permeability of the gut lining which is only 1 cell thick. When this happens, undigested food particles, bugs and toxins from the bacteria themselves can leak through your gut lining into the bloodstream. This wreaks havoc on your body causing inflammation to run rampant. Inflammation is the forerunner to most degenerative disorders and diseases.

If you complain of achy joints, headaches or fatigue soon after eating a meal it may be attributed to a leaky gut. These symptoms may be an immune response to something you've eaten.

Don't take digestive problems lightly. Become a detective and listen to your body. Connect the dots to figure out what foods may be causing you any problems and eliminate them from your diet before matters get much worse.

IMMUNE SYSTEM

The gut plays a major role in the health of your immune system. Sixty to seventy percent of the immune system is located in the digestive track. What takes place in your intestines determines your risk for many illnesses, neurological conditions and degenerative diseases. There are 100 trillion bacteria that live within your gut and these organisms function in a symbiotic relationship to keep your immune system strong. If some of these bacteria are killed off due to eating toxic foods or the overuse of antibiotics, it upsets the whole system.

For instance, when you take an antibiotic, it is meant to kill the bacteria that are causing the infection. Antibiotics should only be taken for bacterial infections and not viruses such as colds and flu. The antibiotic is made to kill bacteria but it does not know the difference between the bad guys and the good guys, therefore, it kills whatever bacteria it comes in contact with. This disrupts the whole synchronized workings of the gut.

Same goes for sugar. Sugary laden foods, artificial sweeteners, high fructose corn syrup and sodas, both regular and diet, are known to be immune suppressors taking a toll on your body. Eating a diet overloaded with this stuff will surely put so much stress on your immune function that you will probably be catching every cold and flu bug that comes around.

Another reason that creates problems for our gut is our Western civilization and our germ phobias. As you can imagine, our gut, with its 100 trillion bacteria, is very diverse. With our western diet, obsession with hygiene, and overuse of antibiotics you may be literally destroying your body's bacterial flora causing drastic consequences to your health. You need all of these bacteria and other organisms living in your gut to maintain your health. Each bacterium and organism has a job to do and we need them all.

In countries where they are not obsessed with hygiene as we are in our country, studies have shown that the microbiome in their guts are as close to that of our earliest ancestors. The organisms in our gut, whether good or bad, are there for a reason. By being overly hygienic, using hand sanitizers constantly, keeping kids from playing in the dirt, etc., we are limiting the diversity of our microbiome and in doing so the gut is no longer able to adapt to what comes along.

My husband's dad used to say; "you have to eat a peck of dirt before you die". I don't think there are many children in our culture anymore who even play outdoors let alone eat dirt! We need the diversity of the bacteria and other organisms in our gut to strengthen our immune system so it can do its job in keeping us healthy. Using hand sanitizers and making everything germ free in our homes is NOT the answer to good health.

Your immune system and your life depend on these hundred trillion bacteria, the inner garden that lives within you.

BRAIN AND MOOD

There is a direct connection from the gut to the brain by way of the 10th cranial nerve. It has long been known by researchers that many mood disorders; depression, anxiety, ADHD, sleep difficulties, etc. can be directly linked to gastrointestinal disorders.

I've also heard of recent research that Autism can be helped by adding certain strains of bacteria to the gut along with a change in diet. I have not had time to do any in depth study at the time of writing this book, but I hope this research is sound. It certainly is exciting!

It stands to reason that by treating gut problems we may very well be treating the underlying cause of many of these mood disorders. Interestingly, 95% of the happy hormone, serotonin, is produced in the gut.

A recent report by the CDC states that depression is the most common type of mental illness, affecting more than 26% of the US adult population. The ADAA, Anxiety & Depression Association of America, reports that anxiety disorders affect 1 in every 8 children. Untreated they are at higher risk to perform poorly in school, miss out on important social experiences and engage in substance abuse. These are pretty scary statistics to say the least.

If you or your children have any mood problems or disorders it may be well worth your while to start eating more nutritious foods (dark leafy greens have the most healing capacity for the gut lining). Eliminate HFCS, artificial sweeteners, flavorings, colors, preservatives and other toxins from your diet and add a good probiotic supplement to replenish the bacterial flora in your "inner garden". See Resource section for my recommendation. Taking these steps first before going for the prescription drugs may make all the difference.

According to Dr. David Williams, "…we can treat the problem from the "bottom up" by repairing the gut and balancing its microflora, without the horrendous side effects associated with psychiatric drugs".

Another interesting connection from gut to brain is the dreaded neurological disorder of

Alzheimer's for which there is no cure as of this writing. In a recent interview with Dr. David Perlmutter, MD, a board certified neurologist, he stated that science is showing that this disorder is directly linked to inflammation.

What is the relationship between inflammation and all the microorganisms that live within our gut? It's the job of our microbiome to regulate the permeability of the gut lining and balance the immune system. Without the proper balance the gut lining (only one cell thick) can begin to leak out certain chemicals and proteins into our body causing an inflammatory cascade that affects the body from top to bottom.

Tons of research is now showing that most of our degenerative diseases, auto-immune conditions and brain and mood disorders are directly caused by inflammation.

This proves the super importance of the gut when it comes to our overall health. Start nurturing the delicate balance of your "inner garden" because it is absolutely critical for your health and life itself.

Baby Steps for Chapter 5

1. Now you know the critical importance your gut plays in your overall health. Become aware of how you feel after a meal. Play the detective role by writing down any symptoms you may have and what foods you consumed. This will help you pinpoint the foods your body can't handle.

2. Get used to reading food labels when you shop. Avoid buying highly processed foods and any packaged foods with High Fructose Corn Syrup. You may want to bring a magnifying glass with you. After all, you are now in detective mode!

3. Start taking a probiotic daily. Take on an empty stomach, usually when you get up in the morning. *In the Resources section I will give you my recommendation for what I have used for 18 years.*

4. Before your meal RELAX just a minute or two. Being stressed while you eat is terrible for your digestion.

5. Stop taking antacids. They soak up the acid that your stomach needs to digest the food you just ate. Instead, figure out what food is causing the upset and quit eating it!

6. Start adding dark leafy greens to your meals to heal your gut lining.

Chapter 6

SUGAR AND PROCESSED FOODS ARE YOUR ENEMY

I know, I know…

I never thought I could live without sweets either!

As I said previously, taking baby steps really does work. I told you how I had been yo-yo dieting for about 40 years and when I started my first diet I discovered Sweet & Low. I thought it was a gift from God since I could have the sweetness without using any of that awful sugar and the calories that go along with it.

As I studied nutrition I realized that these artificial sweeteners are actually worse than real sugar because they are, in fact, chemicals, but did that stop me? NO!

I was a Sweet & Low junkie. Six packets a day and growing. I had it in my coffee and tea, sprinkled on fruit, oatmeal, and anything else that just wasn't sweet enough. I also heard a highly respected nutritionist say that if you have trouble losing weight when dieting it is probably the artificial sweeteners, they're worse than table sugar. Who knew?

I finally had a talk with myself and said that I HAD to give it up. I realized how bad this stuff really was and made up my mind to believe that I would pull it off this time.

I decided to try taking baby steps because I've tried going cold turkey before and it didn't work. I started out by cutting down to a half packet instead of a whole one. Nothing tasted sweet enough but I continued and I got used to less sweetness after about two weeks. Then I cut out the urge to put it on foods that really didn't need it like strawberries. After about three weeks I had gone from 6 packets to 3! Then I started to use just a sprinkle in my coffee instead of a ½ packet. One month later I was Sweet & Low free, hurray! And I have to tell you I do not miss it.

Giving up all sugary foods, not just sweeteners, is your beginning to having more energy, better health, feeling younger and losing fat where you don't want it! As you give up the sugar and add healthy fats to your diet instead, your cravings for sweets will diminish if not go away all together.

Now I can say to you that if I can do it—YOU CAN DO IT. First you have to decide to give up sugar (including foods containing added sugars and/or artificial sweeteners) then you have to <u>believe</u> you can do it and make that commitment to yourself. If you think you can do it cold turkey, go ahead. If that doesn't work take little, bitty baby steps even if it takes a couple of months. Be kind to yourself and feel the success after each step you take (just don't celebrate by eating sugar)!

You will find that it gets easier as time goes by since your cravings begin to disappear. Now read the 5 main reasons below why sugar is our enemy and that should help in your resolve to give it up once and for all.

Why sugar and most processed foods are your enemy:

1. Turns Body into a Sugar Burner (instead of Fat Burner)

Let me start by saying that by eating a lot of sugary foods; sodas, desserts, ice cream and most processed foods, your body becomes a sugar burner. Because your body's metabolism is overrun with so much insulin to process all of the sugar intake, the fat just sticks to all the places you don't want it to.

The good news is that you can, through your eating habits, turn your body back into a fat burning machine as it is meant to be. That means cutting out sugars (and artificial sweeteners) and adding lots of 'good fats' to your diet. Do this and the fat will start melting off without you feeling deprived. See Chapter 7 for more on fats.

2. Compromises Immune System

Sugar is a well-researched immune suppressor. If you find yourself getting sick all the time or catching every cold and flu bug that comes around, eating a diet high in sugar is most likely the reason. Refined sugar significantly impairs the ability of white blood cells to fight germs. If your white blood cells cannot do their job due to your sugar laden diet, this can lead to many other illnesses, including auto-immune diseases.

3. Depletes your Energy

If you lack energy, are tired most of the time or have trouble focusing on the tasks ahead of you, it is more than likely you are eating too much sugar and not enough of the right fats. Your body is meant to be a fat burning machine. Good, satiating fats are precisely the fuel the body needs to produce energy and stop sugar cravings. Good fats are like rocket fuel to your body. You will feel energized and better able to concentrate.

It is true that eating a candy bar (mostly sugar) can give you a boost in energy, a very temporary boost at that, and soon after you are craving sweet. Why? Because sugar is not meant for the body to burn as its source of energy long term. This puts us between a rock and a hard place; if we eat something sweet or drink a soda we may get a burst of energy but after an hour or so we need another boost, and the vicious cycle continues.

4. Contributes to Obesity

As you read above, the body is meant to be a fat burning machine. When we feed it too much sugar and other processed foods it becomes a sugar burning machine. However, once your metabolism is using sugar as fuel, most of the fats in your diet do not get metabolized and are stored right on your hips, butt or stomach. It starts to pile on fast and it seems there is no way out. Low fat diets are not conducive to burning fat off your body either and slowly, but surely, you keep putting on pounds which may lead to obesity. Here is what the CDC (Centers for Disease Control and Prevention) has to say about obesity:

Obesity is a serious concern because it is associated with poorer mental health outcomes, reduced quality of life, and the leading causes of death in the U.S. and worldwide, including diabetes, heart disease, stroke, and some types of cancer.

5. Ages Your Skin (Making you look older than you are)

When sugar or other high glycemic foods such as pasta, bread, chips, white rice, and foods which contain HFCS are eaten they cause rapid spikes in blood sugar levels that release insulin into the bloodstream. This causes a natural process known as glycation. This process forms harmful new molecules called advanced glycation end-products or

AGEs. The more sugar you eat the more AGEs you develop. These compounds prematurely age your body, cause inflammation, and are also linked to other serious health concerns.

Sugar can attach to collagen in the skin and deplete it or break it down. This turns collagen from an elastic, soft substance into a hard, brittle substance manifested as wrinkles and saggy skin.

If these 5 reasons aren't enough to scare you into eliminating sugar and processed foods from your diet then I don't know what will.

Please use this information as a turning point in the way you eat. Knowledge is power. Make the choice now to start cutting out sugars and most processed foods from your diet and that of your family for optimal health. As I mentioned in Chapter 5, excess sugar in the gut may cause leaky gut syndrome which leads to inflammation throughout the body. This sets us up for degenerative and auto-immune diseases, brain and mood disorders, joint pain, and the list goes on and on. Don't set yourself up for a lifetime of illness, fatigue, aches and pains, obesity and so much more.

Baby Steps for Chapter 6

1. Just do a 1% improvement at a time by eliminating one sugar laden food per week.

2. Start eating good fats (more on this in Chapter 7) because they squash the sweet cravings making it much easier for you to do without.

3. Realize that you will never lose fat by eating a diet full of sugars and other refined carbs (no matter how few calories you eat).

4. Buy less pre-packaged foods because almost all of them are loaded with sugar, in some form or another, to keep you buying them.

5. For sugar substitutes use Xylitol and/or Stevia. Stevia comes in powder, liquid or convenient 1 serving packets. I think I've tried them all and the powder and the

packets seem to have a bitter aftertaste but I don't get that from the liquid form. Just try them all and see what tastes best to you.

Chapter 7

MELT AWAY YOUR FAT WITH FAT

Imagine giving up artificial sweetener and now giving up sweets altogether. Guess what? The good fats are so satiating you do not have a craving for sweets! You cannot imagine how good your body responds to cutting out sugars (of any kind). The energy you have is incredible because you are feeding your body the right fuel (good fats).

It is not true that eating fat makes you fat and don't ever believe that for a minute. Your body's energy is supposed to come from the right fuel but when we eat a diet high in refined carbs (sugars and flour) it starts burning those carbs instead. That's when the fat you do eat starts to pack on your thighs and butt because the carbs get burned first.

The vast majority of people in this country are not burning the right fuel, which is fat. They are burning carbs! As mentioned in the previous chapter, the CDC calls obesity the leading cause of death in the U.S. and worldwide, including diabetes, heart disease, stroke, and some types of cancer. Today 2 out of 3 people are overweight!

For decades we have been told to eat low fat diets and look where that got us. There has never been so much obesity and all the ills that come along with it. Why was a low fat diet the cause of the obesity problem?

For one, the food companies compensated for the satiating fats by adding more sugar (in all forms) to their low fat products. This way they still tasted good and of course you thought you were being healthy by eating low fat (not your fault). Secondly, by not eating the good fats you probably didn't have enough energy to get through your day because carbs only give you a temporary boost. So you ate more and more thinking that was what you needed. By now your metabolism is a sugar burner and all the fat just sticks around because your body is using up all its energy just to burn off all the carbs you are constantly feeding it!

Oh what a vicious cycle!

So I am here to tell you that if you simply switch your metabolism to burn the fuel it is meant to burn (good fats) then the fat on your hips, thighs, butt and belly will surely melt off.

You will drop the pounds and the sizes. You will feel full of energy. You will have an overall feeling of wellness. Your joints will stop aching. Your blood pressure will come down. But the best part is that you will enjoy eating this way so much you will never think of it as a 'diet'!

It took me over 40 years of yo-yo dieting to find this out. I have probably tried every 'diet' ever invented. Most of the time I lost a few pounds but it never seemed like I was losing any fat, only the scale would show a lower weight. A few weeks or months later I would gain back those pounds plus 1 or 2 more. So over these 40 some years I put on 25-30 pounds more than my ideal weight. I pretty much gave up on trying another diet when…

I saw this intriguing email about losing fat with fat. After reading it I jumped at the chance to order the program/meal plan because it made so much sense to me. It was digitally delivered to my inbox, I read the Quick Start Guide, the meal plan, made my grocery list and most importantly made up my mind I would give this an honest to goodness try. I told my husband, who had several pounds to lose also, that we were going to try a 'new' way of eating; lots of fats, very little carbs.

He wasn't too happy but I do most of the cooking so he didn't have much of a choice. The first 10 days is what it takes for your body to make the switch from sugar burner to fat burner. It was not hard because everything on the meal plan was so delicious plus it's true what they say…when you eat good fats the cravings disappear!

The first week we both lost 4 pounds, the next week 2 for me and 3 for him. Every week we lost weight and all the time enjoyed eating. There were no cravings for anything. Our lives changed quite a bit after becoming fat burners. Before the 'fat burning diet' we would come home from work every day and just about collapse from fatigue. Now when we came home we were full of energy and felt terrific, no more naps required!

After about 5 weeks we both went down one size. After about 4 months I was down 19 pounds and he was down 20. Plus we both dropped another size. If I didn't do this myself I wouldn't have believed it but I'm living proof that this works. I wouldn't look at it as a 'diet' at all but eating the right foods that our body runs on. This Keto diet plan comes with a Quickstart Guide, meal plans, shopping lists and easy, delicious Keto recipes. If you're interested, I put a link in the Recommended Resources section.

Now if that didn't get you excited there's more. According to Doctor Joseph Mercola, who has appeared on many national television programs such as CNN, TODAY, and the Dr. Oz Show, our body has 2 primary fuel sources: carbs and fats. Fat is the primary fuel source that your body is designed to burn in the most efficient way. When you make the metabolic switch to burning fats you are healing your metabolism at the cellular level. Doing so can *prevent* the development of some of the most common diseases such as cancer, degenerative diseases, high blood pressure and premature aging. Dr. Mercola has just written a new book titled: <u>Fat for Fuel</u> and this is on my 'must read' list.

Some of the best healthy fats you can add to your diet are:

- Avocados

- Coconut Oil (extra virgin organic)

- Olive Oil (if it is 100% all olive) (there is now a scandal about other oils being mixed in with Extra Virgin Olive Oil)

- Butter from grass-fed cows

- Pecans and Macadamia nuts

- Seeds; pumpkin, sunflower, chia, sesame

- Sardines (best source of DHA omega 3)

So please consider making the switch from a carb burner to a fat burner. Remember, fat is the primary fuel source for your body. If you have a few pounds to lose or more than 100 this is the way to do it. If you don't wish to lose any weight make the switch for the sake of your health, to prevent many diseases, gain mental clarity, and increase your energy levels.

I've also recently started a Facebook group, <u>Tips for Keto Lifestyle</u>, where you can get answers to your questions, lots of support and

tons of delicious Keto recipes. Please join me,
I'll look forward to seeing you there.

Baby Steps for Chapter 7

1. Clear out your pantry of industrially processed vegetable oils and hydrogenated oils such as margarines and Crisco.

2. Begin cooking and baking with healthy fats; Coconut oil and coconut milk, extra virgin olive oil, butter from grass fed cows, and others as mentioned in this chapter.

3. Turn yourself into a fat burner to not only lose the fat but to feed your cells what they need to prevent disease.

Chapter 8

STAYING YOUNG
(regardless of your age)

Most of the previous chapters covered a multitude of things that can help keep you healthier and feeling and looking younger. However, I have uncovered so many more ways I just had to add this chapter.

GOOD NIGHT'S SLEEP (Every Night)

A good night's sleep is most important to your health and that of your brain. Our T cells (white blood cells that are an essential part of the immune system) plummet when we are sleep deprived. So if your T cells are low your immune system cannot function as it's supposed to. This, of course, means you are prone to all the cold and flu bugs and whatever else may be going around.

Also, sleep deprivation raises the level of inflammatory markers. As stated in previous chapters, inflammation can lead to all kinds of disease including heart disease, cancer and brain diseases.

I'm sure you have also heard that the body repairs itself as we sleep. Yes, our insides need time to do their thing and that is just what eight hours of sleep provides. So while we are sleeping our body is hard at work completing all of the phases needed for muscle repair and regulating and releasing hormones

During sleep our brain is in its most active state. It clears itself of toxins which accumulate throughout the day. It also releases HGH (human growth hormone) which is the hormone that reduces or prevents many of the problems associated with aging. According to Perimeter Institute eight hours of sleep every night is absolutely necessary to increase HGH release. Just imagine, with 8 hours of sleep nightly, low energy levels, low sex drive, loss of bone mass, and wrinkled skin may become a thing of the past!

I found this most interesting; researchers have recently discovered that our sleeping brains clear out twice as much waste as the waking brain. The waste was identified as beta-amyloid, the toxic substance linked to Alzheimer's disease. If a good night's sleep can protect you from this dreaded disease which has no cure, I'm sure you'll agree that sleeping eight hours a night is worth doing. Be kind to yourself and your brain and give it the time it needs each night to clear itself of these awful toxins. You can be sharp as a tack when your 90!

One last thing on sleep…a recent study involving 1024 participants who habitually slept less than 8 hours a night had a higher body mass index. Lack of sleep can actually be causing you to be overweight. It also disrupts your metabolism because sleep deprivation influences the hunger hormones, leptin and ghrelin. So if you need to lose weight, getting more sleep is a good way to start.

HOW LONG ARE YOUR TELOMERES?

Telomeres are little protective caps at the end of your chromosomes and the length of your telomeres is an indication of aging. Every time a cell divides your telomeres get shorter and once they get too short the cell eventually dies. Shorter telomeres are a sign of aging, on the other hand, longer telomeres keep you younger and healthier. Without testing you really don't know the length of your telomeres but there are certain things you can do to increase or maintain the length of them.

University of Utah researchers have found that subjects taking a daily multivitamin had longer telomeres than non-users. Other research indicates higher intakes of vitamins C and E from foods are associated with longer telomeres. Taking a high quality multivitamin daily could give you longer telomeres thus a longer life.

Another way to increase your telomere length is with the "master antioxidant" glutathione (of which I'm a big fan).

Glutathione is abundant in cruciferous vegetables; raw, steamed or fermented, so be sure to add some to your meals.

You can also increase your glutathione levels by drinking a whey protein shake every day. I have personally been drinking a whey protein shake at least 4 times a week for about 12 years. I don't know what my telomere length is but I do know that I feel 30 years younger than my real age. I also pack my whey protein shake with other good, anti-aging stuff like maca powder (to balance hormones) and blueberries and/or strawberries (anti-aging superfoods). Although whey comes from cows milk and I have totally cut out dairy I allow myself whey because of its benefits. I make my protein shakes with almond or cashew milk and they are so delicious. I find these shakes also keep my energy levels up. I say it's the 'whey' to go.

DETOXIFICATION

I have only done a true detox once in my adult life and didn't realize it was something I should be doing at least once or twice a year. Very recently I attended a class on detox and it really opened my eyes to the utmost importance it has for our health, brain function and emotional wellbeing.

Consider that we come into contact with dozens, if not hundreds of toxins every day. We are 20 times more exposed to toxins these days than a few decades ago.

We breathe them in like fumes from plastics, carpeting and gasoline at the pump.

We eat them with the foods that are sprayed with pesticides especially soy and corn. Also artificial sweeteners, flavorings and preservatives are all chemicals.

We drink them in our tap water which is treated with chlorine (which is bleach) and fluoride and as mentioned earlier in this book traces of prescription drugs are now in most municipal water systems.

We absorb them through our skin with the chemicals in our shampoos, deodorants, makeup, and even wearing permapress clothing. Many of us have a mouthful of mercury fillings which leak heavy metal into our bodies.

As you probably never realized until now, our bodies are bombarded by toxins every minute. Many of our organs function as filters to remove these toxins, however, they just can't keep up. What doesn't get eliminated keeps building up inside. Imagine years and years of toxic buildup inside of you (like a garbage dump)!

No matter how well your kidneys and liver are working they can only process so much. Living, breathing and eating the standard American diet puts our bodies into toxic overload. This causes damage throughout our systems.

What if, once or twice a year, we did a total detox with whole foods, not some fad detox in a bottle. All the systems in our body get a break. The organs can catch up on the garbage pile that's been building up for so long. Your insides are getting a total spring cleaning! Your cells have time to repair, they're clean and fresh and can start rebuilding.

How will you benefit from doing a total detox?

- Joint pain will start to disappear
- Inflammation decreases (remember this is a precursor to degenerative diseases)

- You will feel more refreshed and energetic

- Optimizes your hormone balance and increases libido

- Helps with weight loss

- Clears brain fog

- Improves mood

I'm sure there are many more pluses but the seven listed above will surely help you feel younger. It's more fun to do it with a friend or partner so together pick a time to start and go for it!

STRETCHING and EXERCISING

I know exercising is good for you, however, I must admit I have never, ever enjoyed exercising. One of the best forms of exercise you can do is resistance training.

Your thigh muscles are the biggest muscles in your body and a recent study found that two of the strongest predictors of longevity were strength and muscle mass in the lower body. (*EUR J Clin Nutr 2017;71:64-9*) Exercising these large muscles will increase your metabolic rate, therefore burning more calories. Also by strengthening these muscles you can increase the bone density in the hip and thigh bones, lessening the chance of a severe fracture after a fall.

Doing squats is the best exercise for strengthening the thigh muscles and also the muscles around your hip and knee joints. For the last 15 years I have been working a physical job, climbing lots of stairs and bending and lifting. I guess that makes up my exercise program! But after reading the above study I think I am going to start doing squats regularly.

Stretching is another thing altogether. I love to stretch and very recently started taking a yoga class. I just saw a program on TV that they are now teaching yoga to football players; high-school and pro!

There are approximately 640 skeletal muscles in the human body or 320 pairs. Every muscle constitutes one part of a pair of identical bilateral muscles found on both sides of the body. All of these muscles have a function but if they are never used they become tight and when they become tight we have pain.

Stretching increases the blood flow and circulation to the muscles. This accomplishes several things:

- Elongates the muscles (makes you look younger)

- Straightens posture (makes you look younger)

- Increases your range of motion (makes you feel younger)

- Flexibility (makes you feel younger)

- Muscle tightness relief (makes you feel younger)

- Relieves pain in joints (makes you feel younger)

- Increase in energy (makes you look and feel younger)

- Gives you better balance (makes you feel younger and helps prevent falls)

- Injury prevention (makes you feel younger)

By regularly doing stretching we can feel a lot younger and look a lot younger too! We won't be walking hunched over, have trouble climbing stairs or be unable to reach our upper cabinet in the kitchen. We won't have to worry about falling and having a catastrophic injury. Even if you lose your balance and take a fall, with the muscle strength and flexibility you gained from stretching a major injury is unlikely.

So for all the reasons above and many more—Start Stretching! Take a yoga class or go online and find a stretching program that would be right for you. Just do it!

Baby Steps for Chapter 8

1. Sleep

- Get 8 hours of sleep every night

- Start going to bed at the same time each night

- No caffeine or alcohol before bedtime

- Sleep in complete darkness or wear an eye mask

- Avoid bright light (especially blue light from our tablets) 1 hour before bedtime

2. Telomeres

- Start taking a high quality multivitamin daily

- Make yourself a whey protein shake for breakfast or lunch as many daysas you can (add some anti-aging berries too)

- Add cruciferous veggies to your meals

3. Detox

- If you drink soda, give them up 1 at a time until you've kicked the habit. *(A recent study showed that consuming a 20-oz. soda daily was equivalent to an average of 4.6 years of aging. (Am J Public Health 2014 Dec;104(12):2425-31)*

- Adopt more whole foods into your diet and a lot less processed

- Plan ahead—choose a good time for yourself and find a partner to detox with you

4. Stretch and Exercise

- Find a good stretching program online or join a class

- Check out a yoga class if you never have, you may just love it

- Take at least 15 minutes each day to do some stretching, and add more time as you are able

- Add some squats to increase the strength in your thigh muscles. Do them while you watch TV

PART THREE

FOOD FOR THE SOUL

~~~~~***~~~~~

"Very little is needed to make a happy life; it is all within yourself, in your way of thinking."

Marcus Aurelius
~~~~~

Chapter 9

RELAX FOR A HEALTHY

MIND, BODY & SPIRIT

We need to feed our soul, mind and spirit the same way that we need to feed our body. We need to detox our 'stinkin thinkin' and refresh our thoughts. We need to stop dwelling on the past and move in the present. We need to believe we can have what we desire for our future by taking the right steps in the now.

We can accomplish all of this by taking at least 10-20 minutes a day to just relax, meditate or take a walk in the park. By doing this we put our body, mind and emotions in a peaceful state through which we can become more aware of our thoughts and our life.

In this day and age it seems almost impossible to just take a few minutes for yourself. You carry your cell phone with you at all times. Constant texts are being sent and received, phone calls answered, and of course there's social media. We rarely venture outside except to go from work to the car, the drive home in traffic, then from car into the house. We are busy doing something every second and all this non-stop activity takes a toll on our health. We are basically stressed out and that wreaks havoc on our mind and body.

This is where relaxation or meditation comes in. It is essential to feeling well and living a happy life. We must make the time. Finding 10-20 minutes a day will make your whole life better in every area. Now if you've never meditated before but you closed your eyes and took a nap and drifted off with a smile on your face, that's kind of like meditation. The biggest problem most of us have is quieting the mind that's always worrying, complaining or making problems from nothing.

Here are a few of many ways you can calm and relax yourself:

- Take a walk out in nature

- Color (adult coloring books are a popular craze these days)

- Listen to soothing music

- Soak in the tub and relax to the scent of a lavender candle

- Journal, writing stuff down can be very cathartic

- Meditation

If you choose to learn meditation it will take some time. I have been practicing meditation for about 2 years now and I'm finally able to stay focused for more than 5 minutes. It will finally happen that you can shut off that noisy, sometimes obnoxious, chatter in your head.

Try as many of the different types of meditation until you find the one that resonates with you. Some involve repeating a chant or mantra, there is mindfulness breathing which concentrates on your breath awareness and scanning your body, and there's guided meditation (my favorite), where a soothing voice gently guides you through the meditation. I like the guided meditation best because someone is telling me what to do and my mind doesn't seem to wander as much.

Whatever you may choose to help you relax, it is essential for your health and your sanity. I want to end this chapter with this quote from Buddha when asked what he gained from meditation:

"Nothing, however, this is what I lost: Anger, Anxiety, Depression, Insecurity, Fear of Old Age and Death."

Baby Steps for Chapter 9

1. Set a reminder alarm on your phone (maybe several each day) so you can take 5 minutes or so just to clear your mind and take some deep breaths.

2. Take a nice walk in the park on a beautiful sunny day.

3. Start a journal. Writing down your thoughts, good or bad, helps you cope and relieves stress.

4. Try taking a relaxing bath once or twice a week instead of a shower. Use lavender or eucalyptus Epsom salts which not only scents the water and the air but is also great for pulling toxins out through the skin.

Chapter 10

BE HAPPY!

*"There is no way to Happiness;
Happiness is the WAY"*

Everything we want to bring into our life is for the purpose of making us happy. Think about it…

A beautiful house in the best neighborhood

A career we enjoy that pays a great salary

A soulmate to share our life with

A dream vacation going first class all the way

A healthy body and mind

Yes, all of these would make you happy but you can't precede any of the things you desire by saying, "I'll be happy <u>when</u> I have (any of those things)". You must be happy first.

I can hear you saying "but I live in this tiny little apartment, how can I be happy here?" Well if you want that big, beautiful house you can start by thinking that by living in the tiny apartment temporarily you can be putting money aside for a down payment.

"I hate my job and they don't pay me enough" is another one. While making money at this job you can be looking for another that you will like better and pays more. While searching for that better job you can at least pay your bills.

"I will never find the right person to share my life with" and if that is what you constantly think then you are right. As long as you are focused on <u>not finding</u> your soulmate you won't. What you say and think to yourself is very important in getting what you want. Instead, say something positive like, "wouldn't it be nice if I could meet my soulmate". Keep that in your thoughts and see who shows up!

Same goes for your health. The more you complain about your aches and pains or how little energy you have, and on and on and on, the less healthy you will become. Do not speak or think of how tired you feel or how your joints are painful. Instead imagine how you would like to feel: healthy, full of energy and pain free. Yes, you CAN make up your mind to be healthy and you have just taken the first step by reading this book. Now you have a good start as to how you can prevent many diseases and feel energetic by just eating the proper foods.

The important thing in all of these examples is that if you have negative thoughts (about what you don't want) that's what you'll get. Just figure out a way to say what you want with a positive twist. Thoughts and words act as magnets so you can understand why you want to <u>think</u> about <u>What you Want</u> NOT what you don't want.

I know it's not easy because I only realized this four short years ago. I had to change my whole way of speaking and thinking and there are still times I have trouble turning a negative statement into a positive one. As long as you stay aware of what comes out of your mouth or what thinking is going on in your head you can change. Remember, one baby step at a time will lead to a lifetime of happiness.

Be Happy first while you wait for all of your dreams to come true!

Baby Steps for Chapter 10

1. You must become aware of any complaining and just stop it on the spot. Same goes for any gossiping (very negative).

2. It's hard to be positive all of the time; just concentrate on <u>not</u> being so negative.

3. If you find yourself worrying, remember most of the things we worry about NEVER happen.

4. If you start feeling sorry for yourself, think about all the good things in your life.

5. Be grateful every day for all you do have.

6. When you follow these steps you will begin to see more of what you WANT showing up.

IN CONCLUSION...

If we did everything perfect from the time we were born…

Eat the perfect foods, do the perfect exercises, breathe in perfectly clean air and always be happy, never worrying about anything…

We could probably live forever.

Although that scenario is very unlikely it is NEVER too late to start making lifestyle changes that can help you live longer with better health for your body, mind and soul.

Choose one area of your life that you want to change the most and start there. Use the Baby Steps suggestions at the end of each chapter. Work on just one step at a time, adding another each week or so, and before you know it you'll begin seeing and feeling the benefits.

Take hold of the power within you and use it to stay young, vibrantly healthy and happy all the rest of your days!

RECOMMENDED RESOURCES

<u>Alternatives</u> (a monthly newsletter for the Health Conscious Individual)

I have subscribed to this newsletter since it began.   Dr. David Williams travels the world researching the best natural and alternative cures and I have used many of them. They work!

<u>FAT for FUEL</u> by Dr. Joseph Mercola I am now reading this book and WOW, it is fantastic! His explanations of why we need to be fat burners which not only keeps excess weight off but prevents and/or reverses disease is mind blowing. He also tells you what to eat and when. Check it out.

<u>Brain Maker</u> by David Perlmutter, M.D. This book talks about the rising brain disorders plaguing our country. From Alzheimer's to autism, it may all come down to the health of the gut (your microbiome). A must read.

<u>Enzymatic Therapy—Probiotic Pearls</u> In Chapter 5 I told you that I would recommend the

probiotics I have used for many years. Many probiotics on the market cannot make it to your gut because of the acid in your stomach. These pearls survive the stomach acid. They are very tiny and very easy to take.

Designer Whey Protein Powder This is by far my favorite whey protein powder and I have tried dozens of them. It dissolves easily and it contains a lot more vitamins and amino acids than most others. It also comes in several flavors.

Keto Diet Plan I followed. I would highly recommend this plan as I had checked out several and this one is easy to follow and it works! Here is the link, go check it out... https://bit.ly/2zhMIqV

You can also visit my blog at: http://susangoddardblog.com/

And please come join my Tips for Keto Lifestyle Facebook Group at:

https://www.facebook.com/groups/tipsforketolifestyle